Yoga for Everyone

Yoga for Everyone

✦

Helping to make the world a more centered place, one person at a time.

April Farrell-Hasty, RYT

Visit my Web sites
www.lotuslore.com
www.innerpeaceyoga.org

iUniverse, Inc.

New York Lincoln Shanghai

Yoga for Everyone
Helping to make the world a more centered place, one person at a time.

iUniverse books may be ordered through booksellers or by contacting:

iUniverse
2021 Pine Lake Road, Suite 100
Lincoln, NE 68512
www.iuniverse.com
1-800-Authors (1-800-288-4677)

ISBN-13: 978-0-595-35924-0 (pbk)
ISBN-13: 978-0-595-80378-1 (ebk)
ISBN-10: 0-595-35924-8 (pbk)
ISBN-10: 0-595-80378-4 (ebk)

Printed in the United States of America

Intention

The intention of this book is to be a brief introduction to yoga and some of the accompanying concepts. It contains practical information on how to clean your yoga mat and other questions you may have had but did not ask.

It will serve as a reference guide for you to add your own wisdom, so, when you go to yoga class, workshop, or a weekend intensive, you can bring this book and use it as a resource or add to it. It is intended for new yoga students.

Introduction

At the center of your being you have the answer;
You know who you are and you know what you want.
~ Lao-tzu ~

It's not what happens to you,
It's what you do about it.
Taking responsibility for change.
~ W. Mitchell ~

Encountering sufferings will definitely contribute to the elevation of your
spiritual practice, provided you are able to transform calamity and
misfortune into the path.

~ H.H. the Dalai Lama ~

What is yoga to me?

If you have chosen to read this book you are trying to improve your life. And I
am the QUEEN of improving my life, so you have chosen wisely. Changing any
aspect of your life takes courage, discipline, and a true desire to change. Yoga has
that effect on people. You add yoga to your life and, you stop eating foods that
are bad for you, stop smoking, _____ (fill in the blank). Yoga creates
positive changes.

Every culture has some ancient tradition that is unique. For example, Tai Chi,
Chi Kung, Karate, Krav Maga, and yoga to name a few. What is unique about
yoga is it is aerobic, (depending on the style you choose) weight-bearing—you lift
your body weight; it increases flexibility, decreases stress, and is readily available.
Yoga is a natural movement that is easy to learn. You need no equipment to do
yoga. (Although equipment is often be helpful.) Yoga is old (over 4,000 years),
mystical, and very misunderstood. Yoga is a therapeutic way to heal the body of
painful afflictions. Yoga can also heal the mind. It is a moving meditation and
some asanas (poses), headstand for example, can ease depression, help a headache,

and improve memory. All of this from headstand! Yogic breathing can improve asthma, bronchitis, and pneumonia.

I have a hereditary illness, sickle-cell anemia, and yoga has done so much for me. I could spend two days discussing the benefits I have received from yoga. I have come so far. B.Y. (before yoga) I thought I built a wing in the hospital near my home with all my frequent visits. I was so sick! I would be in the hospital for two weeks, get out, go home for a few days, and be admitted again for another two weeks. I lived like this for years while traveling with the military, with two small children and a husband who was patient and loving beyond belief. I stand corrected this was not living. It was a painful existence. A.Y. (after yoga) I rarely get hospitalized! I once went five years without hospitalization. I still got sick during this period. I either stayed home, went to the doctor, or I went to the emergency room and went home in a few hours. This improved the quality of my life 150 percent. This is how I currently live. I still have bad days, but they are few and far between.

I have done yoga for many years—most of my life actually. But I never really practiced yoga until I was in my late 20s. I did asana, not much pranayama or meditation.

When I put it all together I practiced yoga and this is when the changes occurred in my life. I could not connect to the spiritual side of yoga at first. I was confused. I did not know where I belonged spiritually. Most of my 30s I read every religious book I could find. I read the Bible, Upanishads, Vedas, Koran, and several other books. I could tell you about being a Sikh, a Quaker, Taoism, Hinduism, and Scientology. I was seeking a reason for my illness, why was I born with a hereditary illness? Why was I so sick? Why, why, why me?

I read Louise Hay, any book on healing, I became a Reiki master. I also became a lay doctor, as a military wife I often moved places where I was the only sickle cell patient. I could tell the ER staff what I needed in their terminology. Some military doctors had never encountered a patient with my illness. I can read and understand my chart like a doctor. I can read medical shorthand, and I learned the valuable skill of firing a doctor while sick lying in the bed. I was seeking an answer. And like most people I had the answer in front of me all the time. I realized it was not about me. It was what I had chosen to experience.

I would not trade B.Y. for A.Y. for any amount of money. This is not an endorsement that yoga can cure sickle cell anemia or any other illness you may have. This is what yoga and lifestyle changes have done for me. I rarely see the doctor now. I went from seeing my hematologist every four weeks to seeing him every twelve to sixteen weeks for a CBC (complete blood count) to check my H&H (hemoglobin and hermatocrit). I now see the acupuncturist and the massage therapist more than I see the allopathic doctor.

I have seen arthritic people feel better with yoga and not be as stiff. I have seen kids with ADD calm down. I have seen elderly people attend yoga class and make friends in class where once they were isolated and lonely couch potatoes. This is not a scientific study although they do exist. This is just my personal experience.

When I do yoga solitary it feels mysterious and like a familiar old friend. I also find that when I practice yoga alone I sometimes get lazy and do not push myself as I would with a teacher. With a teacher yoga feels new to me, as I am experimenting with new poses and learning the way I do a pose is sometimes slightly out of alignment—it is a learning experience still after all these years. I never want to become complacent and think I know all about yoga and think I don't need to take a class. I take a class once or twice a week and will continue to do so.

> Better to do something imperfectly
> than to do nothing flawlessly.
> ~ Robert H. Schuller ~

This book came to be as a result of my writing a first book for yoga teachers. I began to think students would enjoy one as well. With practical information and also basic introduction to a few yoga principles in an easy-to-understand manner with concise instructions. (I did not want to overwhelm the new yoga student and chase you away!)

My background in yoga is diverse and different. My husband retired from the Air Force. During the time prior to that, we moved every two to three years. I would move to towns that had no yoga, or very little. Most places had Iyengar so I took a lot of that. But I also took Kirpalu, Integrative Yoga Therapy, Viniyoga, Phoenix Rising, Anusara, Jivamukti, and the list goes on. So I would study IYT (integrative yoga therapy) and move someplace where there was no IYT and start Jivamukti, for example. (Two very different types of yoga.) I tried to get certified for a long time, (12 years) but we moved before I could finish anything. I finally completed my training in 2002 and became a RYT (Registered Yoga Teacher from Yoga Alliance) after my husband retired. Now when I look back I realize I had a comprehensive education studying everything for two years. The problem was I needed to know more about a style before I could commit to studying it. When I finally decided to study it there was not enough time to complete the training.

Acknowledgments

In our daily lives, we must see that it is not happiness that makes us grateful, but the gratefulness that makes us happy.
~ Albert Clarke ~

I get by with a little help from my friends
~ The Beatles~

I wrote this small book and it was an overwhelming undertaking. I literally said one day, I am going to write a book. I sat down and wrote an outline and started typing. It is good to be naïve otherwise this book would not exist. If I knew how difficult it was to write a book I would have never done it. I am an avid reader and I assumed it would be easy. It was a blessing that this book was the first book I wrote. I started writing a much larger book on a different subject and instinctively I put that book aside to write this smaller book.

Have you ever heard the saying it takes a village to raise a child? It takes a village to write a book? Thank-you to my husband for being a photographer, being photographed, and being patient. Thanks to my family for their support.

Thank-you to the staff of iUniverse. Thanks Kerry, my editor who held my hand and made a difficult job easier. She was so patient and kind. Thank you to Jan for being photographed for the photos in this book, Thank you, Rich for being a photographer and a good friend. Thank you, Vickie Hasty for your organizational skills.

Again Ron who has always supported me no matter what I do.

Irene Hasty, my mother-in-law, author of two books, who supported me in this process. My children, Bryttani and Arjay, for their kind words when I was frustrated. Thank you, Mom for your help.

A special thank-you to the staff of Yoga Alliance and Sandy Van Oosten for use of the Students Bill of rights. So I dedicate this book to all the people who helped me and believed in me.

I also took classes and workshops with well-known yoga masters. I thank you for your wisdom. But they already have lots of recognition.

And to all those teachers I had on the road as a military wife. They all helped me more than they realized. Here are a few that helped me so much. They made such an impact on me and were so inspirational.

Pamela Viviano–Viniyoga, White Lotus
Judy Day–Integrative Yoga Therapy, Phoenix Rising Therapy
Nancy LaNasa–Jivamukti, Shivananda
Maggie McClain–Hatha
Vaz Rodbeck–Hatha, Ashtanga, Iyengar
Saravati Devi–Hatha, Ashtanga, Iyengar
And to all those I have yet to meet.

Thanks to all my students, I have learned the most from you. All my students have taught me about yoga, about myself and my character, and more importantly about being a yoga teacher. And teaching any subject it is about what is best for the student. I gratefully acknowledge my students contribution in molding me into the teacher I am today. Thank you to all...I prostrate gratitude and love.

Om shanti
April

What Is yoga?

Yoga comes from the Sanskrit word *Yuj*, meaning "to yoke." Yoga means union. It integrates the body and mind. We often treat the body and mind as two distinctly different things; yoga integrates the body as one by using asana (poses), pranayama (breathing techniques), and meditation—balancing body and mind. Creating flexibility in the body and in the mind. Yoga is the union of mind and body.

How Yoga Came to the West

Swami Vivekananda came to the United States in 1893 to teach Raja yoga in Chicago. He was exotic and different, and several well-known thinkers and writers were stimulated by his different way of thinking and viewing the world. In the 1940s, Russian-born Indra Devi came to Hollywood and had several famous students. In the 1960s, the English musicians, The Beatles studied transcendental meditation with Maharishi Mahesh. The counterculture of the 1960s brought yoga and meditation to the forefront; other celebrities, such as Madonna, Gwyneth Paltrow, Sting, and Willem Dafoe, have more recently helped to expand its practice.

Benefits of Yoga

Physical Benefits
Increases flexibility
Improves balance
Adds length and strength to muscles (tones the muscles)
Can be done regardless of age
Stimulates the digestive, nervous, endocrine, and circulatory system
Helps maintain joints and the spine by increasing lubrication to joints
Enhances the immune system
Decreases stress and moderates hypertension
Massages the organs of the body
Flushes toxins out of the body
Improves breathing; helpful for people with respiratory problems
Lifts the derriere to give you "yoga butt"
Can be used to help mild back pain
Can be helpful in weight reduction
Increases energy level
Builds strong bone helping with osteoporosis

Mental Benefits
Improves stress
Self-awareness
Headstands or legs up the wall pose can be used to help in mild depression

There are many more benefits of yoga.

The Importance of a Good Yoga Teacher

When I am out and about, for example, at a social function, the conversation inevitably turns to "What do you do?" When I say I am a yoga teacher, I hear every story imaginable about yoga. But the thing I hear most often is "I do yoga to a video." My response is "Where is your teacher?"

Most people feel a video is enough. I tell them a good teacher will keep you from doing harm to yourself. There are rules to yoga, and unless you know them and have had instruction over time, your body may be harmed for lack of instruction. This makes no impact. I guess we yoga teachers might see these people after the damage is done. I tell them to do yoga in front of a mirror in their bedroom to see their form if they have no intention of going to a class. The problem I see most is that the student does not know *proper form*. People frequently ask me, "Isn't yoga performed alone?" I say, "Yes, it is after you've learned the basics." You would not drive a car without instruction; why would you harm your body doing yoga without instruction? A few of these people have come to my class. I think to learn proper form is easier than to unlearn incorrect form. It is difficult to see your form, even if you have a mirror; as soon as you turn your head to look in the mirror your form has changed.

Yoga Students Bill of Rights

By Yoga Alliance
www.yogaalliance.org

This information is provided by Yoga Alliance.

Thank you, Sandy Van Oosten and the staff at Yoga Alliance.

Short Version:

As a Student I have the right to uphold my own values and integrity at all times. If they are compromised or challenged in any way, I have the right to clearly state my values and know the Yoga Instructor will respect them. If I am not respected, I have the right to investigate and act to ensure my values, standards and personal ethics are upheld.

Long Version:

Yoga is about union—on a personal level. When you first begin a yoga class, you will be exploring new ways to breathe, move your body and challenge your flexibility. The journey begins with creating safety for your body. The longer you practice yoga, your awareness shifts from the external safety to an inner journey of "ways to breathe, move your body and challenge your flexibility." You may begin to challenge your energetic, emotional, mental and spiritual security.

As you read the guidelines, be willing to allow the "rights" to expand from physical safety to an honoring of the sacred, personal aspects of your life.

Yoga does not equal asana (posture) on just the mat—but asana all of my life. As I practice within a classroom, I realize I may experience inner, emotional openings as well as physical challenges. To honor and respect the all levels I am exploring, I have the right to:

~ be in a safe and sacred space.

~ adapt asana and practices to allow for personal safety on all levels. This may include having an opportunity to ask questions appropriately.

~ compete with myself, not the expectation of the teachers or others in the classroom.

~ request not to be assisted.

~ Only be touched in a safe and sacred manner.

~ be spoken to and treated respectively and with loving kindness by the teachers and students in the class.

~ expect confidentiality of anything shared in a classroom.

~ establish healthy boundaries for my practice—anatomically, emotionally, mentally and spiritually.

~ be challenged to explore my therapeutic edge.

~ be allowed and encouraged to be in my inner journey, not just the physical aspect of the practice.

~ stay in integrity and uphold my values at all times.

This is reprinted by permission of Yoga Alliance. "Yoga alliance registers both individual Yoga teachers and yoga teacher training programs that have successfully demonstrated compliance with the minimum educational standards established by the organization."

From www.yogaalliance.org

How to Find a Yoga Teacher

Since yoga has become so popular, it is everywhere. Gyms, at the park, recreation centers, and, last but not least, yoga studios. Most yoga studios hire qualified teachers, *although that is not always the case.* A lot of people are certified in weekend programs. Truly qualified teachers spend years becoming qualified. I spent years, and earned a 500-hour teaching certificate. Five hundred hours with a focus on anatomy versus a weekend class that took 20 hours—which would you prefer?

I teach in both a yoga studio and a gym. In the gym I substitute a lot. I don't have a class of my own, but when I teach there the students love it. Unfortunately, they are unwilling to go the studio and pay more than what they already pay at the gym. By the way, the people I substitute for have only 20 hours of training, and their classes are not the same as taking a yoga class in a yoga studio (which is only my opinion). I have taken their classes out of curiosity. Recognize the difference between real yoga and fitness yoga. Fitness yoga is generally taught in a health club. Don't get me wrong, several qualified yoga teachers teach yoga in health clubs, but most prefer a yoga studio atmosphere. And unfortunately the students *don't* know the difference when it comes to the quality of the class. The yoga done is not always safe in health clubs. If you are not being corrected, the teacher is not teaching you by correcting improper form. If the teacher is doing the entire class (every pose) with the students, how can she or he help you? If the teacher is not using Sanskrit, this is a good indication of how well the teacher is trained. Most good teacher training schools emphasize Sanskrit. Ask the teacher whether they are certified and, if so, through which organization or organizations. Determine whether the Yoga Alliance or The British Wheel of Yoga recognize it. If they are not certified, ask them whom they have studied with and for how long. If they are certified through fitness certification only, ask how long their certification took to acquire and how many certifications they hold. You have a right to know whether the person knows what they are doing before you follow them and risk injury to yourself.

There are a few good teachers who, for whatever reason, are not certified. I have a good friend who is dyslexic and cannot take the exam or write the papers, but she has over twenty years of experience and is a wonderful yoga teacher. I suggested she take an oral exam, and she found someone willing to give her one.

For more information on yoga certification or to find a teacher, please visit the following Web sites:

www.yogaalliance.org, Yoga Alliance
www.yogateacherassoc.org, California Yoga Teachers Association

I wrote the following article because students often ask whether they can lose weight with yoga.

"The Yoga of Weight Loss"

The question I am asked most is "Can I lose weight with yoga?" The answer is yes. Any exercise at all is better than being sedentary. A great thing about yoga is that it increases flexibility, which can be very important as a person gets older. Face it: no one is getting younger. But choosing the yoga that is right for your body type is not always easy. Yoga can make you feel stronger. There are as many types of yoga. The problem is that new students find it difficult to find a class that matches their current activity level. What do you like? What is your current exercise level? How active are you? What I recommend varies for each individual, but what follows is a basic reference guide.

If you currently work out a couple of times a week, try a Hatha class.

If you work out to qualify for the Olympics, try Ashtanga (very vigorous aerobic class).

If you don't work out at all, you ought to try gentle class for a beginner.

Choose the level that is appropriate for your current fitness level. Your teacher can direct you to the appropriate class for you. Check with your physician if you have any medical problems before beginning any new exercise program.

I always recommend a basic class for newcomers. Yes, if you are an athlete you will probably be bored, but at least you know that in advance it may not be as difficult as you would have liked. But if you choose something too difficult it is my experience that students do not come back. Yoga is then labeled too difficult. Yoga works your muscles in different ways than other exercises. Also, in yoga you lift your body much like in a push-up. So if you are used to pumping iron, it will be a big shock when you discover you are unable to stay in a pose. The ability to do other exercises like lifting weights, for example, does not necessarily mean you can do yoga well on your first attempt. Do not be surprised that yoga is more difficult. I have taught professional football players, bodybuilders and even they were amazed how much effort yoga was.

Yoga is about having fun. It's not serious. As my teacher likes to say, "There are no yoga emergencies." Have a good time, enjoy the class, and be open to new challenges. Yoga may seem strange and wonderful. Be prepared for shavassana (relaxation translated into corpse pose). At the end of many yoga classes there is a relaxation period for the last ten to fifteen minutes of class. Enjoy it. I have seen so many new students uncomfortable with just letting go and relaxing. Why is it so difficult to relax? Just be prepared for it and try to let go of all your thoughts.

The following is practice for weight loss designed to work the digestive system (check with your physician first, please):

- Surya Namascar (sun salute) A & B four times each
- Trikoasana (triangle) each side twice
- Parsvakonasana (side angle) each side twice
- Parvitti Trikosana (revolved triangle)
- Parvitti Parvokoneasana (revolved side angle)
- Ardha Chandrasana (half moon pose)
- Parvitti Ardha Chandrasana (revolved half moon)
- Vrksasana (tree), Garudasana (eagle), Eka Pada Utkatasana (one leg chair)
- Shavassana

Repeat the entire practice twice. But please work up to two times consecutively. This is not a very time-consuming practice, but it is slightly challenging. After a few weeks, add a few asanas.

Also be prepared to be sore after you have stretched muscles. Soak in Epsom salts after class, or use your favorite muscle rub. You will be surprised how much it helps.

Last but not least, remember that you can lose weight with yoga, but you need to do yoga consistently (a few times a week) and watch what you eat. Make sure you have chosen the correct class for your abilities. Keep a food diary. Weight loss is a simple formula. Expend more calories than you take in. Be patient with yourself. It took a while to gain weight; it will take a while to lose it.

Guidelines for Beginners

Here are the rules for beginners before you go to your yoga class.

Before you go to class

Research which class is best for you.

Don't eat for the two hours before the class—I have had students eat a full meal and become ill.

Don't wear any fragrance to class. Students come to class smelling like they walked through a car wash of perfume. It is overpowering and offensive and some people are allergic.

Be on time—get there fifteen minutes early. New students may have to fill out paperwork (e.g., release forms, next of kin in case of emergency, etc.). It is rude to show up late and have the instructor stop class to get you situated, when everyone else was there on time.

Have cash—not all studios accept credit cards. Also tell the teacher any illness or medical problems you may have, as some asanas (poses) should not be done in certain medical conditions. Call the studio ahead of time to find out if you need anything other than a yoga mat. Ask if they have extra mats to borrow. (Most studios do.) You may need a block, blanket, or strap.

Once you arrive at the studio

If asked, remove your shoes before walking into the classroom/studio.

Under no circumstance should you ever walk on anyone else's mat! This is the personal space of others and should be respected. They may put their faces on the mat. Step over the mat to get where you need to be, or walk in front of or behind the mat.

Your teacher may accidentally step on your mat to adjust you, but most teachers will try not to.

Go to a class that is appropriate for your fitness level

If you have never taken a yoga class, take a beginning class. If you do not work out and are overweight, ill, or out of shape, take a gentle class. If it is too easy, next time try a beginner class. I have had students in my class complain that it was too difficult. Yes, it would be if you were unaccustomed to exercise and have chosen a class that is too difficult for your current fitness level.

Know your limits. Do not push your body. I give alternatives to each pose but new students, for whatever reason, tend to be competitive in my experience and want to keep up with everyone else. Some of you will inevitably choose the more difficult option at your peril.

Come to class in a good frame of mind, ready to learn. Try to handle criticism well. Teachers may touch your body or comment on your actions. This is intended to be helpful to you. And don't give up. Come back to class regularly. That is how you improve in order to enjoy more fully the benefits of yoga.

Wear loose-fitting clothing. Some students have come to class wearing jeans. I always wonder whether they wear jeans to the gym. You need to have a free range of motion, and restrictive clothing can only hinder your experience.

Don't compete with other students! Yoga is not competitive. You do not know how long the other person has been doing yoga. You, on your first day, cannot compete with someone who has been doing yoga for a year, so why try?

Prenatal

I have had third trimester pregnant women come to a nonpregnancy class because someone told them, "You should go to yoga." I turn them away at the door. I am capable of teaching pregnant women, but they are limited by their size and what they can do by the trimester they are in. That's not fair to the rest of the class. I usually give them the information for the pregnancy class.

Get your doctor's approval to practice yoga.

Get referrals from your doctor for prenatal teachers.

Talk to other yoga students who have children and get referrals from them.

Talk to yoga teachers; inquire about good prenatal teachers.

Once you have chosen a teacher, ask for references and credentials.

Are you comfortable with this teacher?

The teacher should ask for your doctor's approval, what exercise routine you had prior to pregnancy, how far along you are, which pregnancy this is for you, and whether there are any complications.

Choose a class that fits your level of fitness. If you did Ashtanga (challenging yoga) prior to your pregnancy, would you be bored in a gentle class?

Do not attend class if you are not feeling well.

Dress comfortably, and wear a bra with very good support.

Drink plenty of water before, during, and after class. It is important to stay hydrated.

Avoid extreme twisting and lying on your stomach; lie on your side.

Stop if you experience chest pains, uterine contractions, or vaginal bleeding.

Enjoy class!

Meditation

Meditation is quieting the mind. All day long you have so many thoughts. Just to still the thoughts and simply be can be difficult to do at first, because your thoughts will not stop. With time and practice it will become easier. Most yoga centers offer meditation. Try it a few times before you judge it. Keep an open mind.

To start a meditation practice:

- Choose a time when you are not in a hurry. Most people do it in the morning.

The rishis (sages) meditated at 3 AM. I must admit I do it at 6 AM.

- Meditate at the same time daily.
- Sit facing east. It is supposed to give you more energy from the Earth's magnetic field, which is said to improve your meditation.

Meditation Retreat

If you are a beginner to meditation you need to perhaps read a book or look online for more information before deciding on a retreat. Before any meditation retreat or workshop, investigate the credentials of the teacher, talk to the teacher to find out the style that is taught. Is the style compatible with you? If you are used to simple breath counting (counting your breath to 10 and starting over if a thought interrupts your counting) a Zen meditation would be very difficult.

Choose a retreat that fits your level; why attend a residential retreat when you can sit for a day workshop? If you are new to meditation a residential retreat would be difficult, choose a day retreat.

Bring a *zafu* (meditation cushion) or comfortable pillow or ask if you can sit in a chair if needed.

Bring water, tissues, and cough drops if you need them.

Enjoy your sit!

Who's Who of Yoga?

Yogi Bhajan gives yoga information freely that at one time was very secretive and forbidden to give away. He started the 3HO organization. He practiced Kundalini and was the Mahan Tantric until his death in 2004.

Krishnamacharya learned yoga from his teacher Rama Mohan Brahmachari in a cave. He was a scholar and a householder (married, with children). He taught at the royal palace in Mysore, where he trained Iyengar, Sri Pattabhi Jois, Indra Devi, Mohan, and several others. What is astonishing is that Krishnamacharya had so many students who went on to create dynamic styles of yoga, such as the men listed hereafter.

Iyengar was Krishnamacharya's brother-in-law and was very ill. Eventually he cured himself of several illnesses. He was very sick as a young man.

He later went on to create a style of yoga based on alignment, and is well-known for curing people of various ailments. In his book *Light on Yoga* there is information on various ailments.(And how to improve them.)

Pattabhi Jois taught at the Maharaja Sanskrit College in Mysore, became a professor, and retired. He tours the world teaching Ashtanga. He is almost ninety years old.

There are many more masters of yoga.

Types of Yoga

Different ways to reach enlightenment. The first four types are what all yoga is divided into. For example, Hatha is Raja yoga.

Bhakti—Yoga of devotion to a god or guru. Selfless love.

Raja—*Raja* literally means "king." Royal path yoga meditation-based eight limbs. (Eight limbs is the path of a Raja yogi) can be found in the yoga sutras 2:29-30.

Karma—Yoga of selfless service involves selfless service (seva)—think Mother Teresa.

Jnana—Scientific approach. Who am I? Inquiring about the self.

Iyengar—B. K. S. Iyengar, of Pune, India. Deals with alignment of the body, uses props (blankets, blocks, and straps). Nicknamed furniture yoga.

Anusara—Means flowing with grace. Graceful yoga, alignment with loops of the body, it is said if you practice Anusara you cannot harm yourself. Headquarters located in Texas and created by John Friend. And throughout the world.

Hatha—Sun and Moon
Ha—Sun
Tha—Moon
Hatha is an umbrella term for yoga. Several different types of yoga are considered Hatha.

Ashtanga—Originated by Sri Pattabhi Jois in India. There are 241 poses done in 6 series. This should only be your first class if you are a serious athlete. It is said that Pattabhi Jois's grandson, Sharath, is the only person on Earth doing the sixth series. Very aerobic yoga, you must first do the primary series, secondary and each series becomes harder and more challenging.

Bikram—Twenty-six poses done in a heated room with mirrors. Also known as Hot Yoga, located in Beverly Hills, California, and throughout the world.

Integrative Yoga Therapy—Meditation, affirmation, healing-focused yoga. Located throughout the world.

Jivamukti—Founded by David Life and Sharon Gannon. *Jivamukti* means "liberation while alive." It focuses on chanting in Sanskrit, learning yoga literature, and the asanas. Located in New York City and throughout the world.

Kali Nata Yoga—Ma Jaya Sata Bhagavati, founder of Kashi Ashram. Awakens Shakti in us all. It involves kirtan during asana, and turning inward. The main yoga center for Kali Nata Yoga is in Atlanta, Georgia, with Ma Jaya in Sebastian, Florida, and throughout the world.

Kundalini—Yogi Bhajan, a Sikh, told the secrets of this yoga so all could utilize it. Raising serpent energy from the first chakra upwards. Founded the 3HO (happy, healthy, holy) foundation, makers of Yogi Tea.

Kiripalu—Meditative and spiritual focus on inner life and releasing long-held emotional blocks. Kirpalu center is located in Lennox, Massachusetts. Taught throughout the world.

Siddha—Gurumayi Chidvilasananda is the founder, and Swami Muktananda brought it westward. Looks at divinity in everything to seek enlightenment. Vedanta, system of philosophy in the Upinashads that reality and a self-identity is towards a single goal. Ashrams throughout the world.

Sivananda—More meditative approach using the eight limbs. Ashrams throughout the world.

Tantra—Tantra means weave. Teaches that spirituality is everywhere and in everything. Yogi Bhajan was the Mahan Tantric. (He left his body in 2004.)

White Tantra—Releases subconscious blocks and karmas. Deals with balancing polarity. To practice you must be in the presence of the Mahan Tantric to transmit the energy. Yogi Bhajan of Kundalini yoga was the Mahan Tantric. He died in 2004 and a new Mahan Tantric at the time of this writing has been chosen. To practice tantra find a tantric or kundalini teacher.

Red Tantra—Basically, two people are moving energy as one person tries to move up the chakras, and attain bliss on Earth. White and red tantra most popular. Although it is not as sexual as you might think. It does not always involve the sex positions in the *Kama Sutra*.

Viniyoga—Krishnamacharya's son, Desikachar, and grandson, Katsub, carry on the tradition in India. Viniyoga adapts the pose to suit the individual's needs to whatever they may be.

Yoga Warnings

~Inversion Warnings
    (Headstand, handstand, shoulderstand, and legs up the wall)
    Do not do if you have:
    High blood pressure
    Detached retina
    Menstruation

Pranayama Warning
Before practicing pranayama warm up first with gentle breathing.

Ask your teacher about your particular situation.

How to Select Your Yoga Mat

Most students choose the most inexpensive mat they can find, which is fine, but if they choose to continue yoga, they are usually not happy with this choice. I have seen students put two mats together to make it more comfortable. I have one large, heavily padded mat. And this mat is what I recommend for students, just because it is comfortable, more comfortable than two mats together. Buy your own mat; do not use borrowed studio mats. Most are cleaned on a regular basis, unless you are cleaning it when you are done. And they clean them on a daily basis. I know of students who got foot fungus at a studio I taught at when I first became a yoga teacher seventeen years ago. It was traced to the mats that were borrowed.

How to Wash Your Mat

Yes, you need to wash your mat. You sweat; there are germs. You lie on it and put your face on it. Walk around the studio barefoot.

I have had lots of people tell me they wash their mat in the washing machine. I personally have never done this, nor would I. Students also tell me they never wash their mat. I clean my mat on a monthly basis, sometimes more, depending on the situation. And I have twenty mats, travel home, a thick mat for workshops, one for teaching, and so forth.

I recommend that you lay it on the floor and fill a small spray bottle with warm to hot tap water and five to eights drops of tea tree oil (tea tree oil is a strong antiseptic). Spray the mat, leave it on the mat for forty-five seconds to a minute, and wipe it off. Flip it over and do the other side. I also use a few drops of sandalwood oil to make it smell less antiseptic. I then let it air out for a couple of hours.

Yoga Vocabulary

Acharya. A guru, one who has mastered yoga

Ahimsa. Non-harming, nonviolence, first yama. (Raja yoga path in the yoga sutras 2:29-30)

Asana. Seat, poses, third limb of yoga

Ayurveda. Science of life, form of medicine using doshas (body/personality types). Ayurveda comes from the Vedas, a book as older than the Bible with information on how to stay healthy. Ayurvedic practioners follow this advice to have maintain health.

Bhakti. Yoga of devotion to a god or guru

Bodhi. Enlightenment Buddha, awakened one

Chakra. Wheel, energy center along the spine, head, above the head, etc.

Dharma. Truth, teachings of Buddha; in Hinduism, it means moral duties and responsibilities

Dristi. Focus, gaze

Guru. Spiritual teacher

Karma. Law of reaction, based on the Vedas and the Upanishads, your actions determine your destiny in your next incarnation; the sum of your actions determines your future existence

Three Types of Karma

Karma created now, in this life, experienced in this life
Karma created now, in this life, experienced in the next life
Karma created in this life but experienced after several lifetimes

Karma yoga. Yoga of action, to do for others without your needs being met (think Mother Teresa)

Kosha. One of five sheaths that cover the self (Atman)

Kumbuka. Breath retention, to hold and direct the breath. It is said you are not practicing pranayama if you have no kumbuka.

Kundalini. Coiled serpent energy present at the base of the spine

Mahabharata. Ninth century BCE Sanskrit epic of civil war between the Pandavas and the Kauravas in the kingdom of Kurukshetra. The *Mahabhrata* is a very important book in Hinduism.

Mantra. *Man* means to think, *tra* means "tool" or "instrument"; mantra literally means "tool of thought"; mantras are phrases, symbols, and religious words that are repeated for a chosen period of time to bring about a desired result; some are to attract a mate, others to bring wealth, but most are for spiritual purposes.

Namaste. "I humbly bow to you." *Nama* means "bow," *as* means "I," and *Te* means "you"

Om. The vibration/sound that created the universe in Hindu cosmology; a common mantra

Patanjali. Individual who organized the yoga sutras; prior to his organization, the sutras were passed by oral tradition, from teacher to student; Patanjali was said to be a physician

Prana. Life force, energy, chi

Pranayama. Breath control Prana = breath, energy, yama = restraint, also referred to as breathing in yoga. But it actually means breath control.

Raja Yoga. Royal path of yoga as referred to by Patanjali

Rishi. Vedic sage, title of a master

Samadhi. Bliss, eighth limb of Patanjali's path, becoming one with the universe

Sanskrit. The classical language of India; language yoga is written in; yogic asanas are often called by Sanskrit names

Shakti. Feminine power, consorts of deities

Shiva. Deity, male power, god of destruction in Hinduism

Sutra. "Thread," as organized by Patanjali

Tantra. "Loom," tantrism, spiritual evolution using the feminine form; Hatha yoga comes from Tantra

Yoga Sutras. Teachings of yoga organized by Patanjali

Yogi/Yogini. Someone who practices yoga

Jan is demonstrating the asanas below. Here is her bio.
You're never too old for yoga. Jan took her first yoga class in her mid 50s and at
69 is a massage therapist and a Certified Yoga Instructor working with seniors

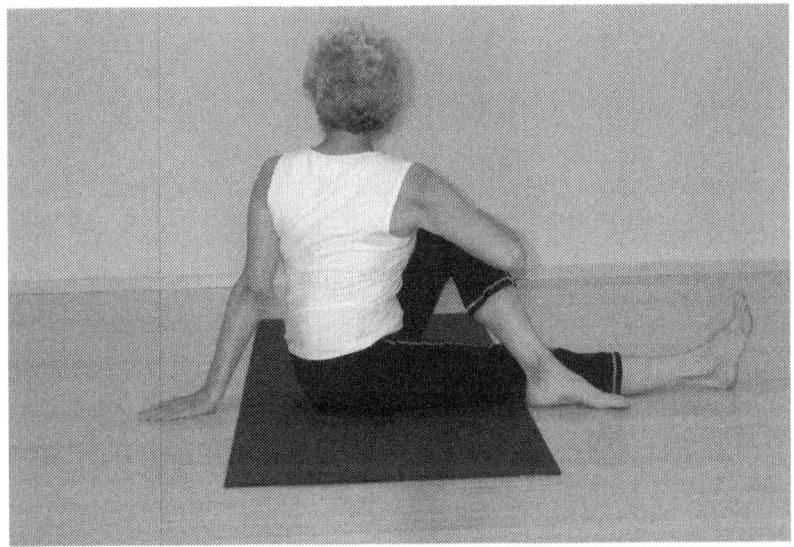

Seated twist

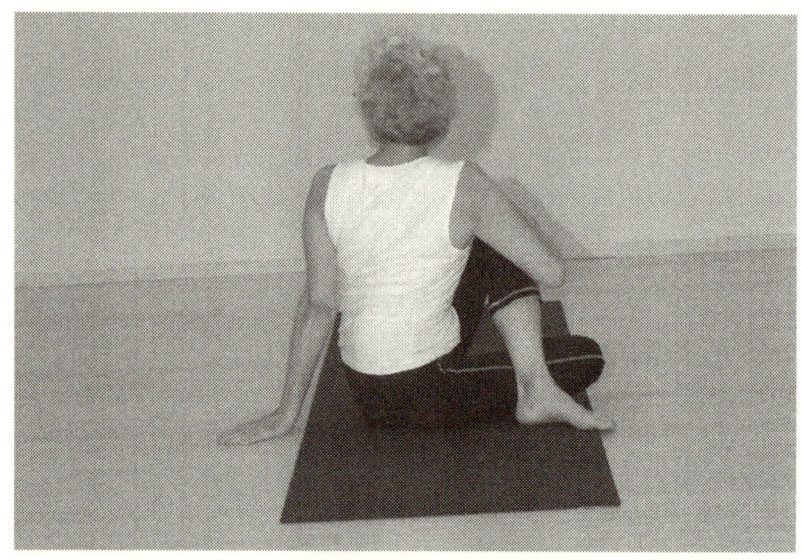

Seated twist different view

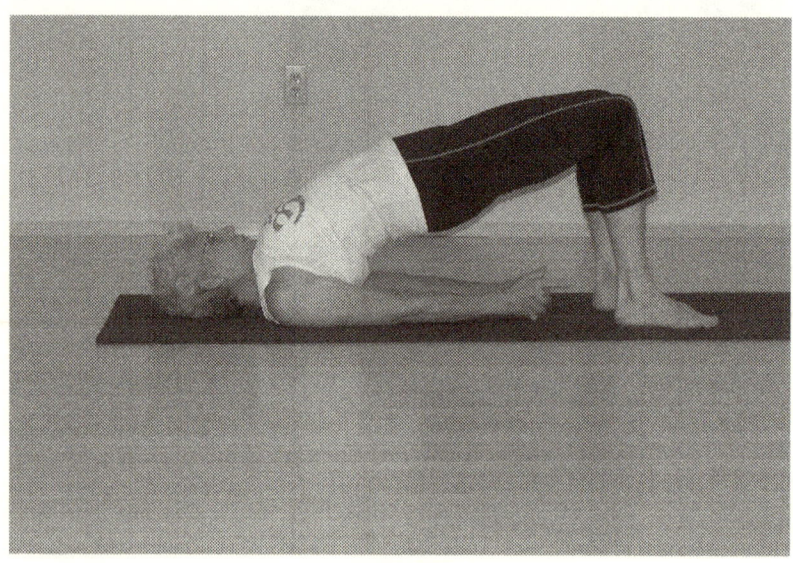

Bridge
Setu Bhanda

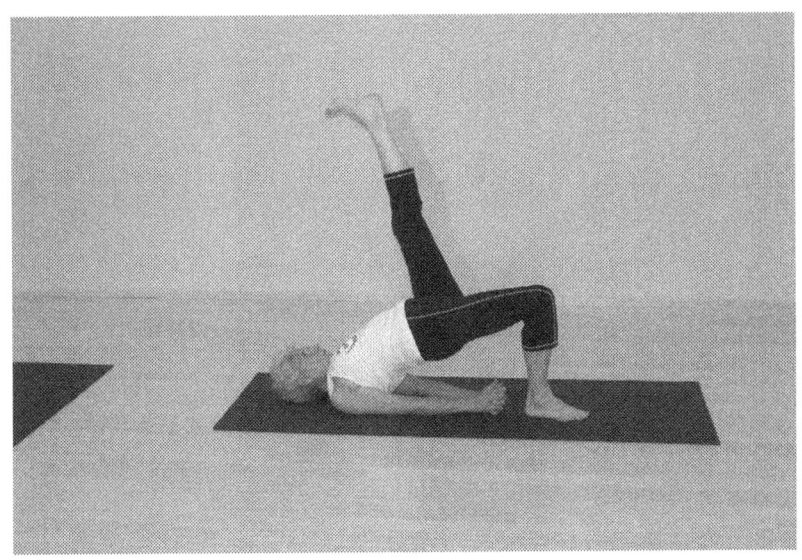

Bridge with one leg up

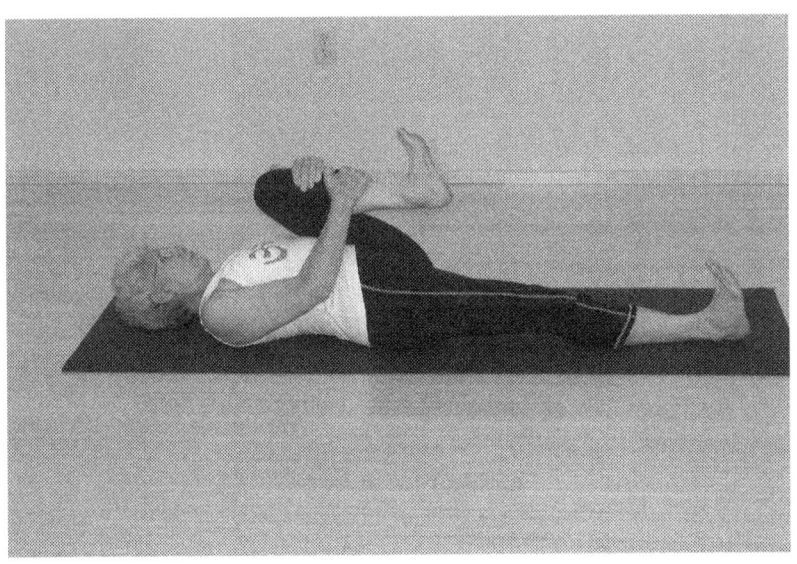

Knee to chest

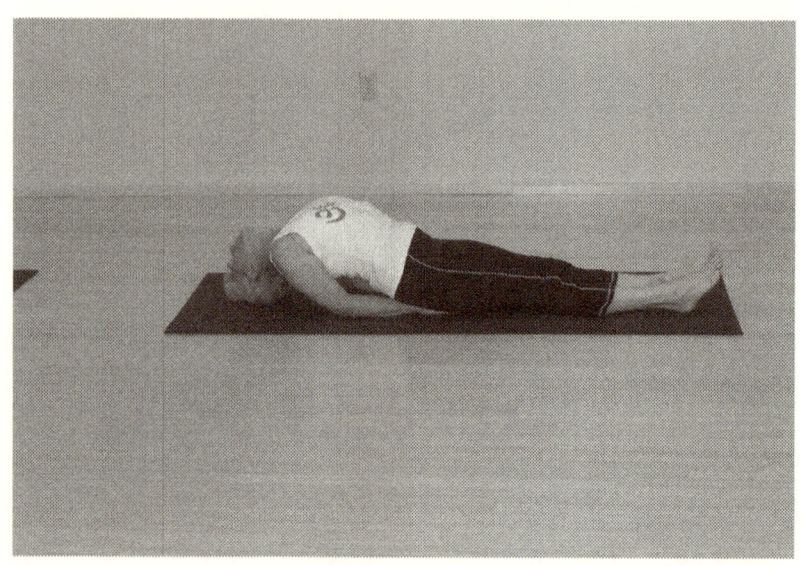

Fish
Matsyasana

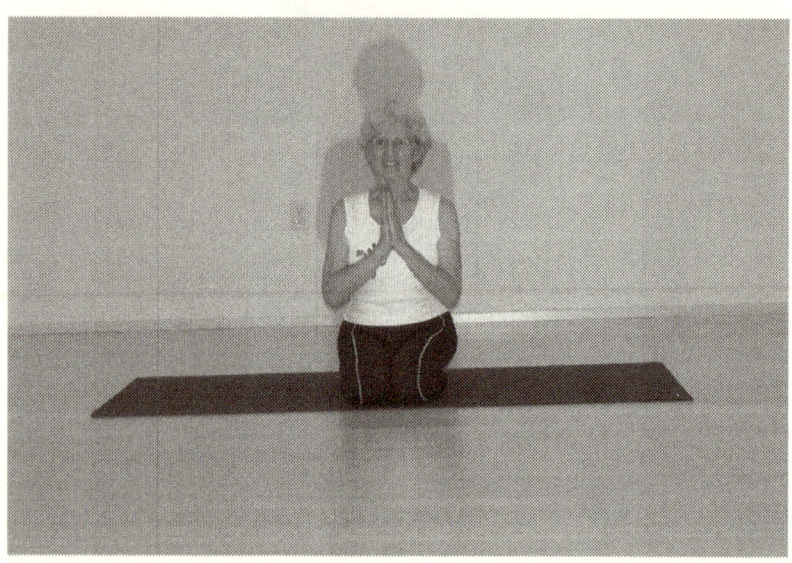

Hero
Virasana

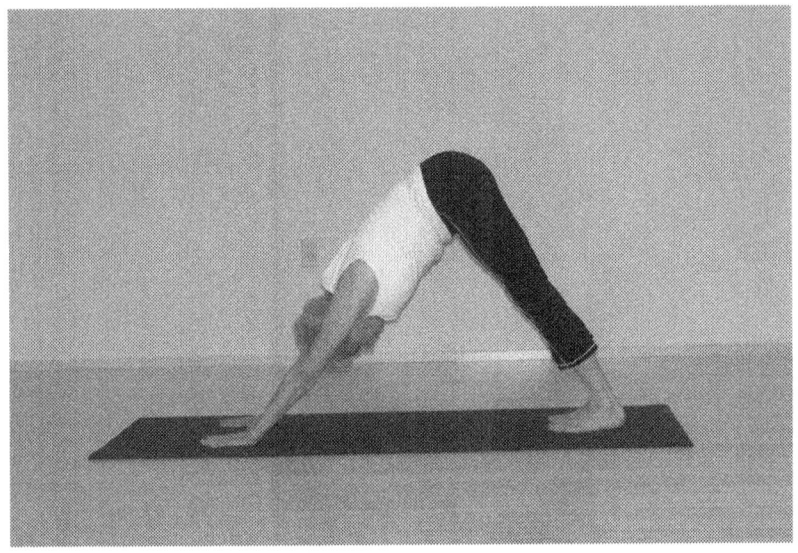

Downward Facing Dog
Adho Mukha Svanasana

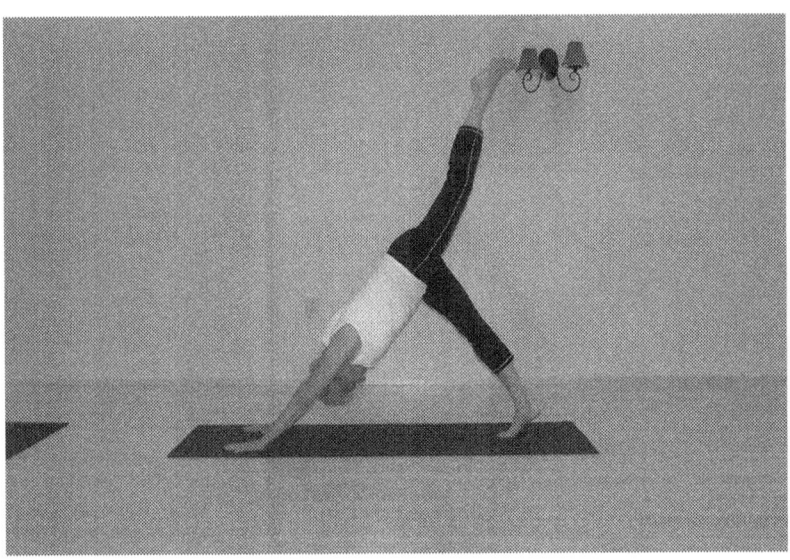

Downward Facing Dog with one leg up
Eka Pada Adho Mukha Svanasana

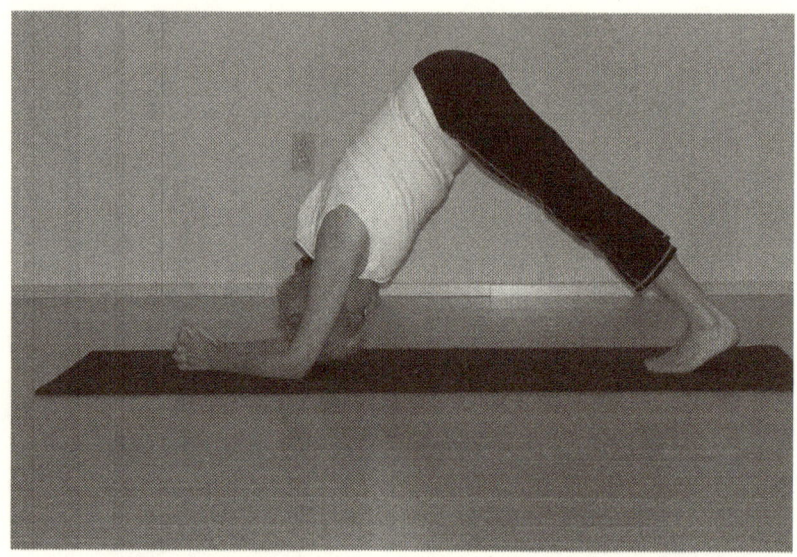

Downward Facing Dog elbows down often referred to as Dolphin
Adho Mukha Svanasana with elbows down

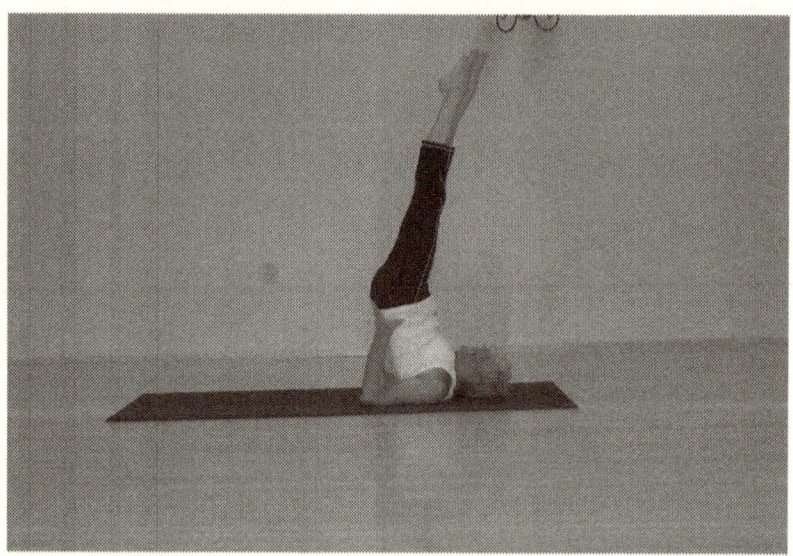

Supported shoulder stand
Salamba Sarvangasana

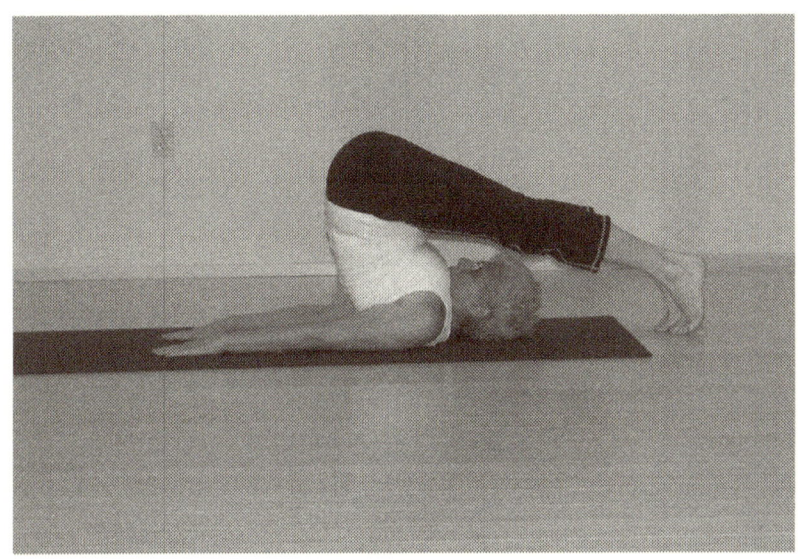

Plow
Halasana

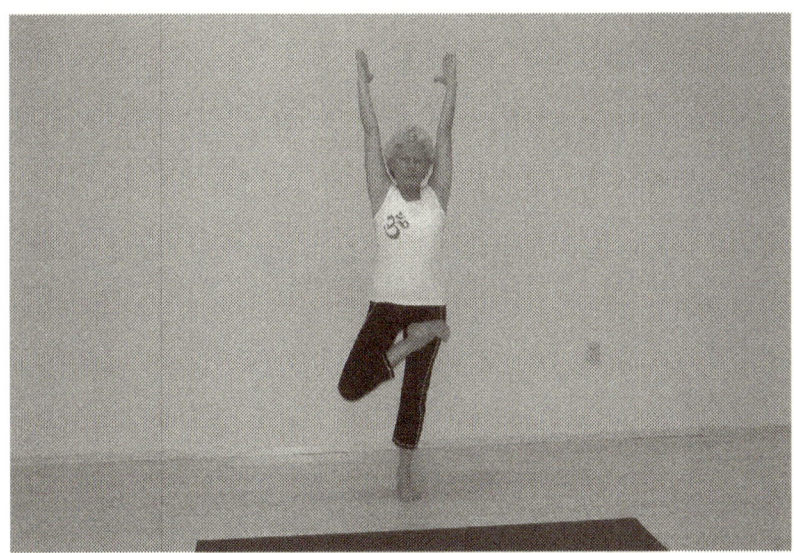

Tree variation
Vrksasana

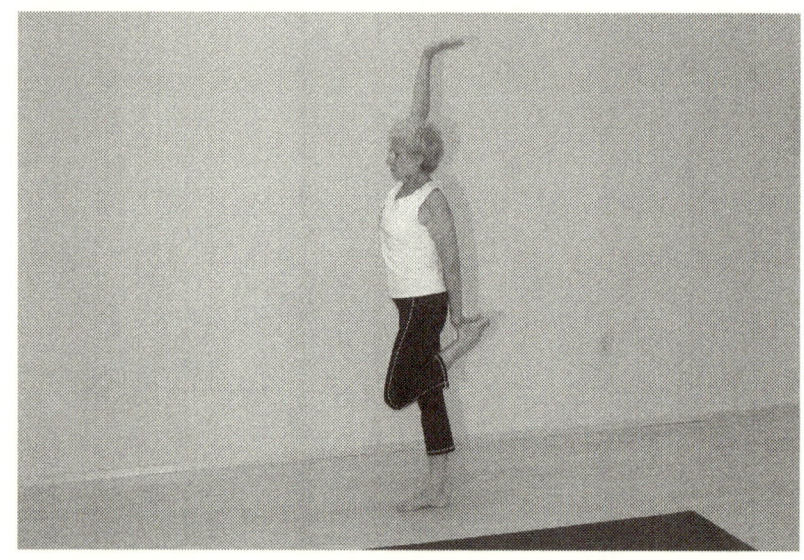

Dancer prep
Natarajasana

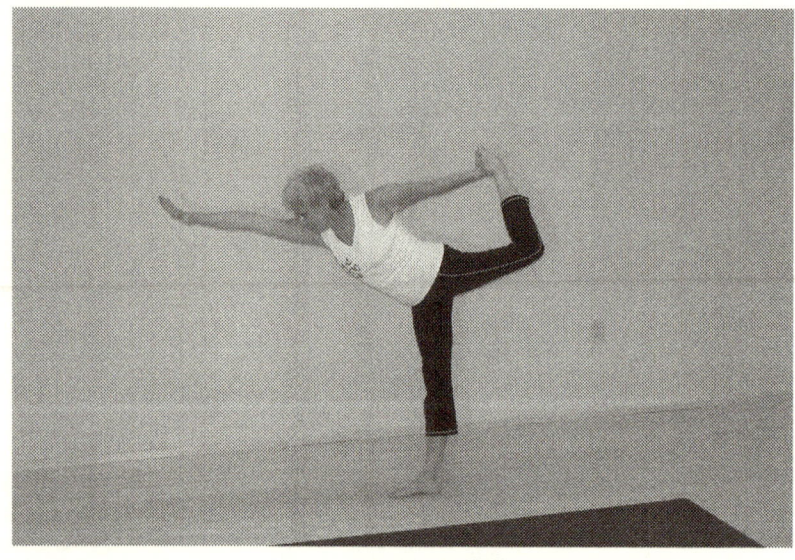

Dancer
Natarajasana

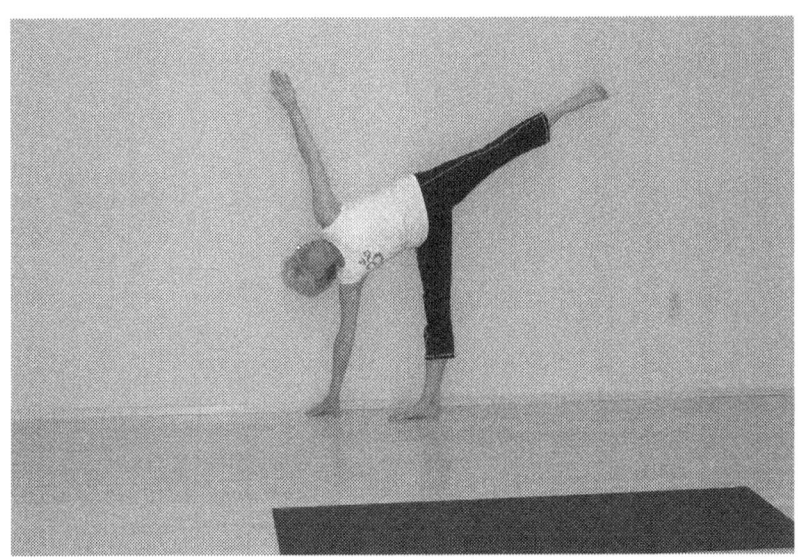

Half-moon pose
Ardha Chandrasana

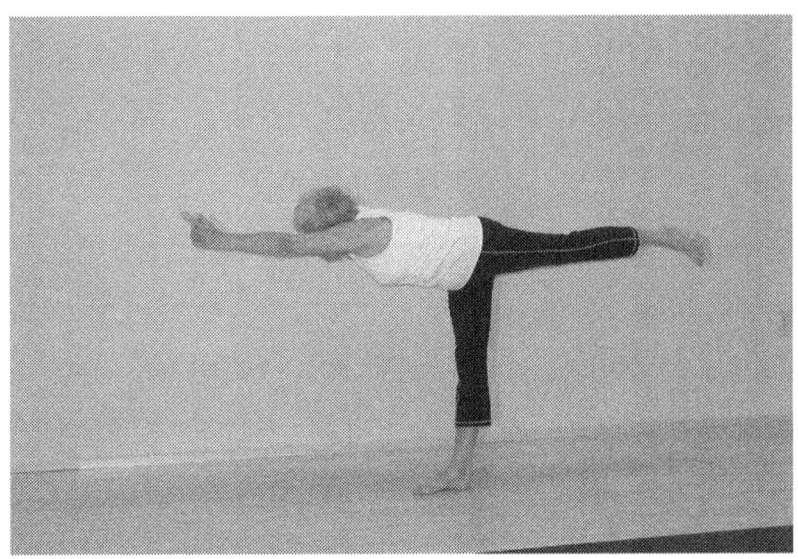

Warrior III
Virabhaadrasana III

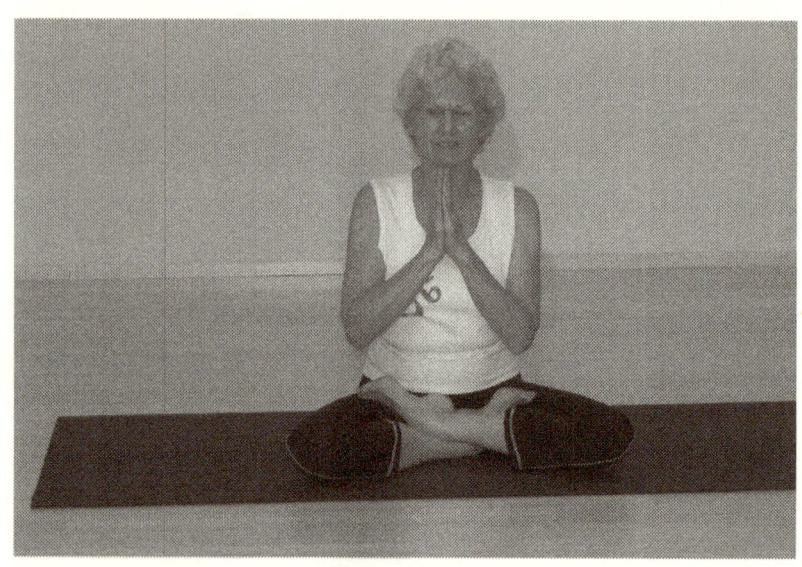

Lotus
Padmasana

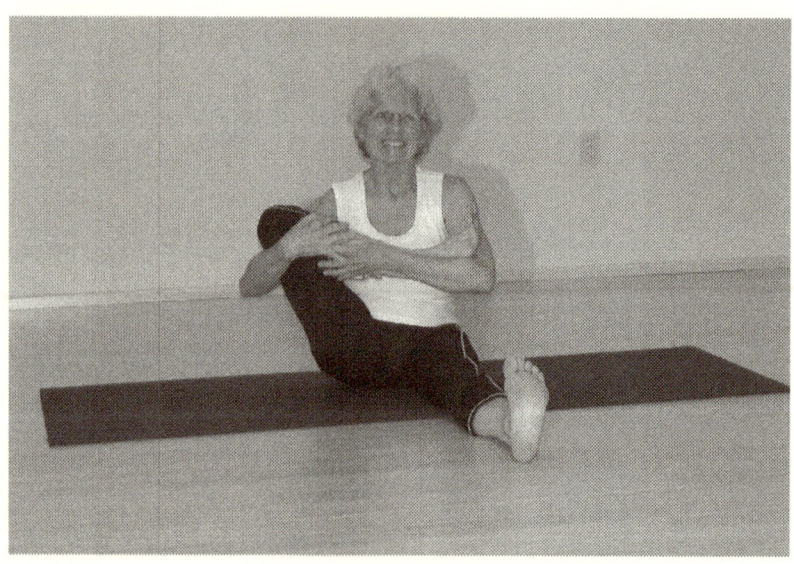

Leg behind the head prep

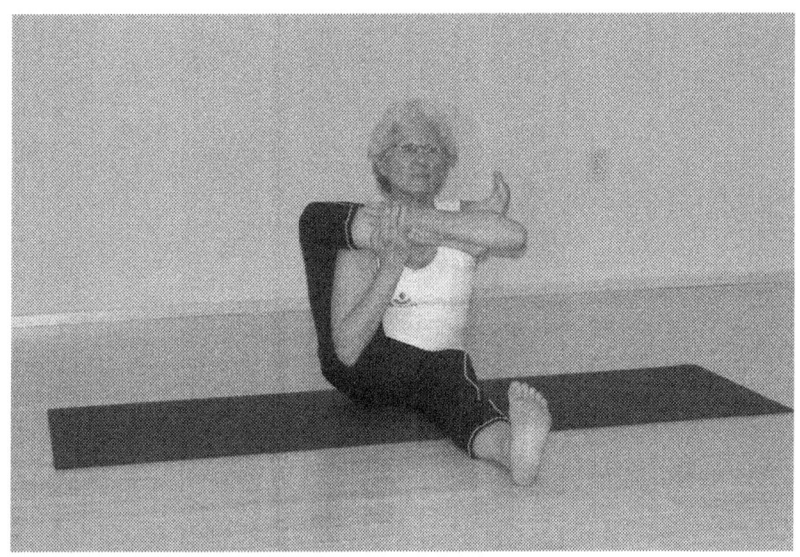

Leg behind the head prep

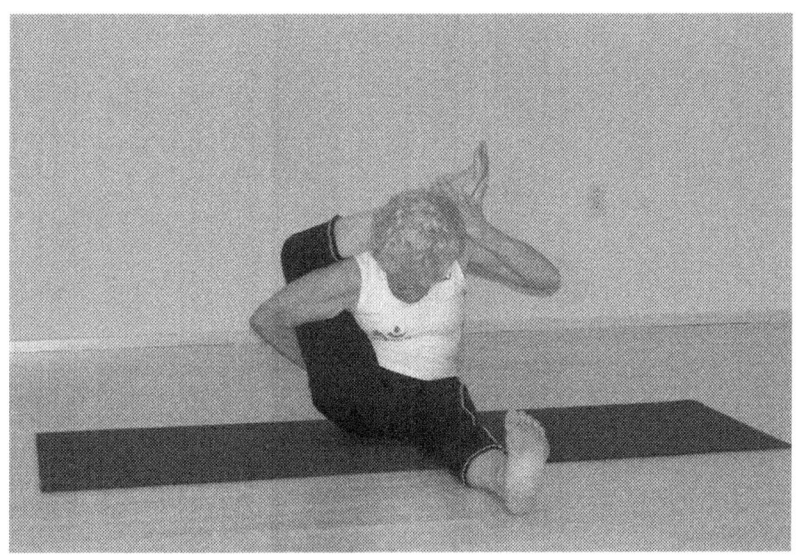

Leg behind the head

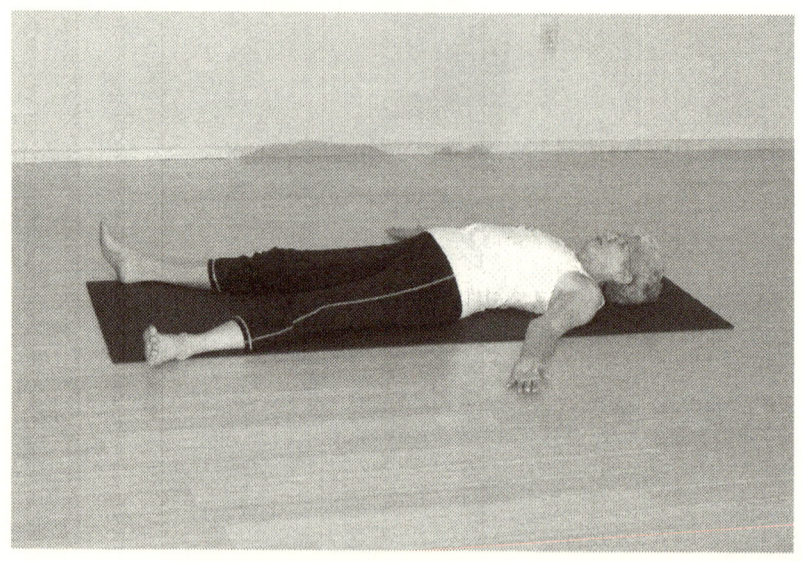

Corpse pose
Shavasana

Ron came to yoga as the result of being rear-ended in a car accident. Yoga has improved his injuries.

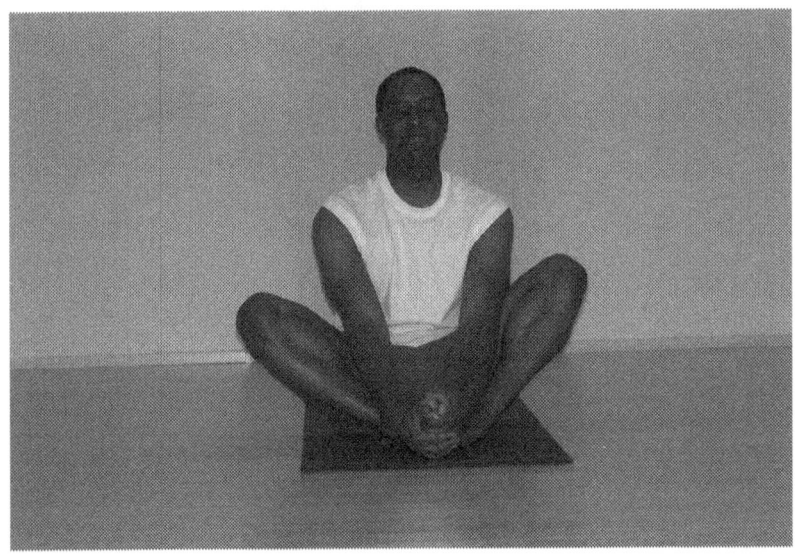

Cobbler's pose
Bhanda Konasana

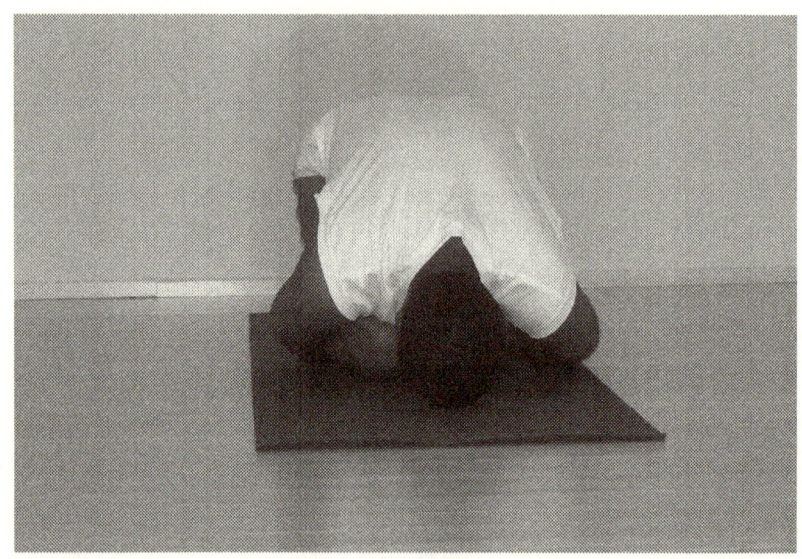

Child's pose
Balasana

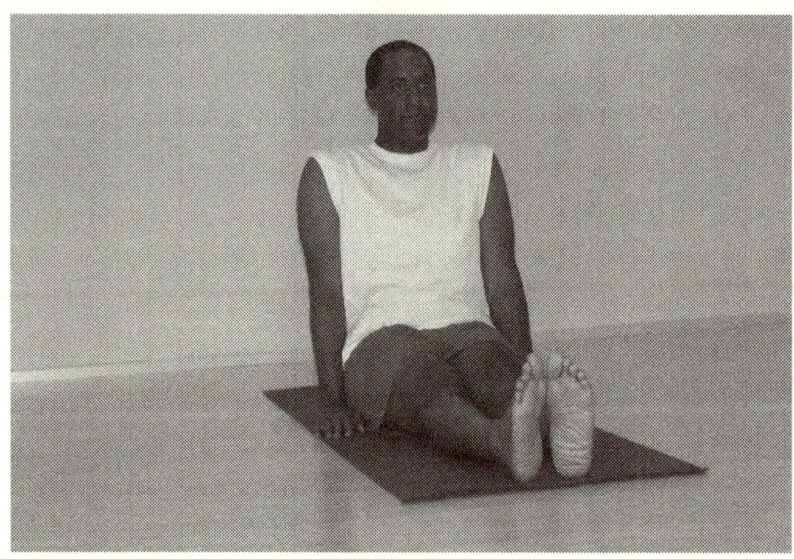

Seated four limb pose
Dandasana

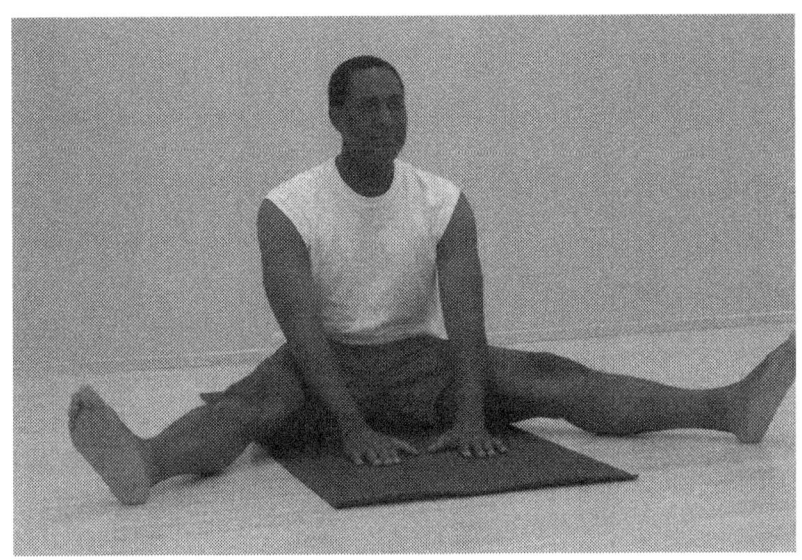

Legs wide

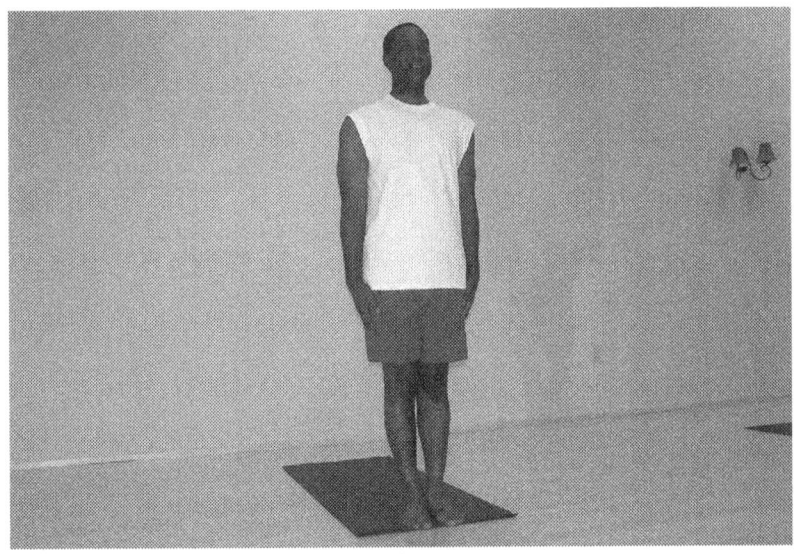

Mountain
Tadasana/Samasthiti

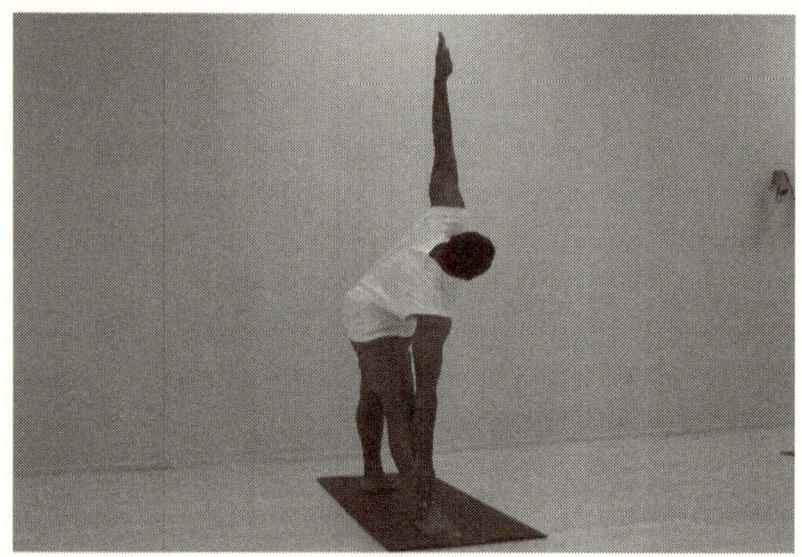

Triangle
Trikonasana

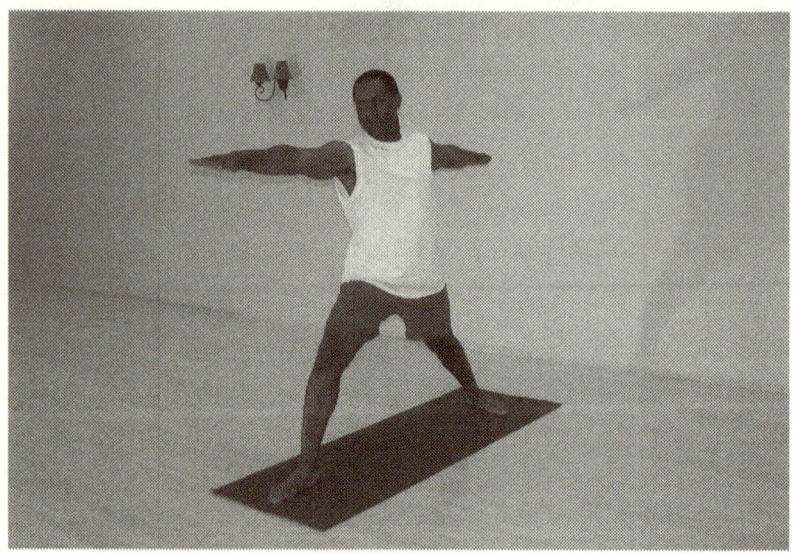

Warrior II
Virabhaadrasana II

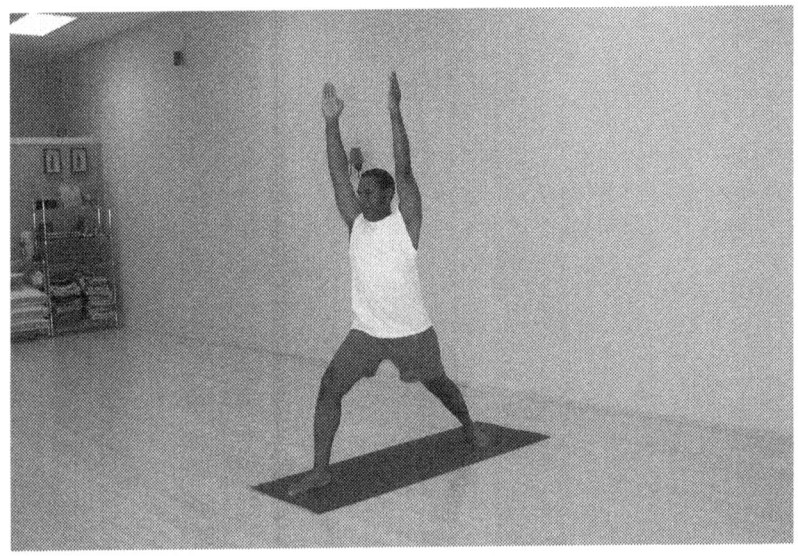

Warrior I
Virabhaadrasana I

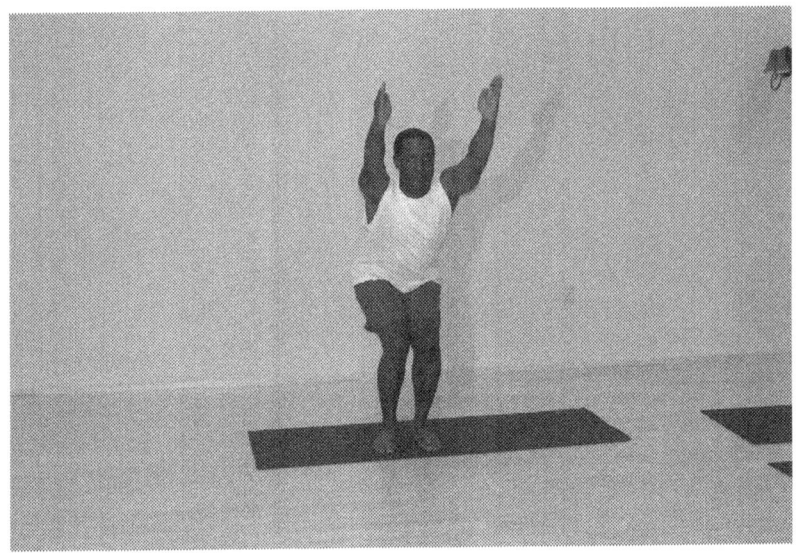

Chair pose
Utkatasana

I purposely put in my book photos that show me not doing the asana perfectly. My legs are not perfectly straight, but I am not injuring myself. I used this image to show yoga is not about perfection, it is about enjoying the journey. And the journey is a magical one.

Sometimes we are overly concerned with alignment we no longer enjoy the journey.

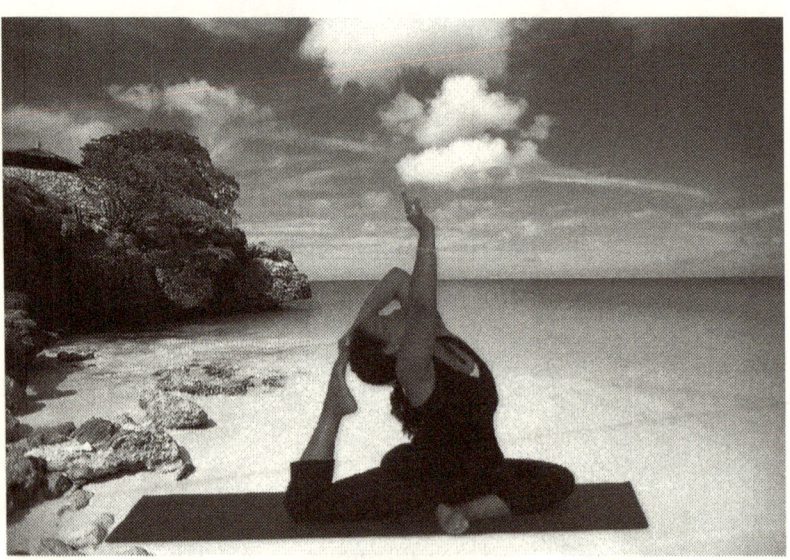

One leg king pigeon
Eka Pada Raja Kapotasana

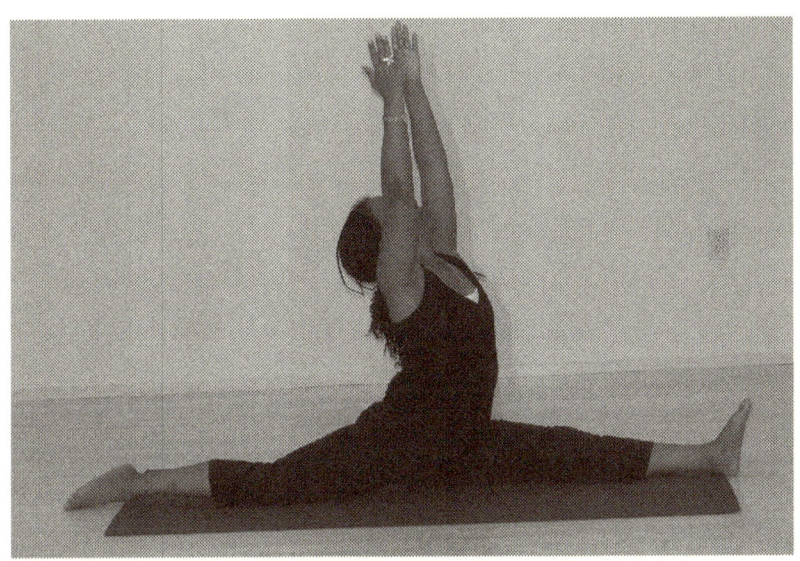

Split
Hamumanasana

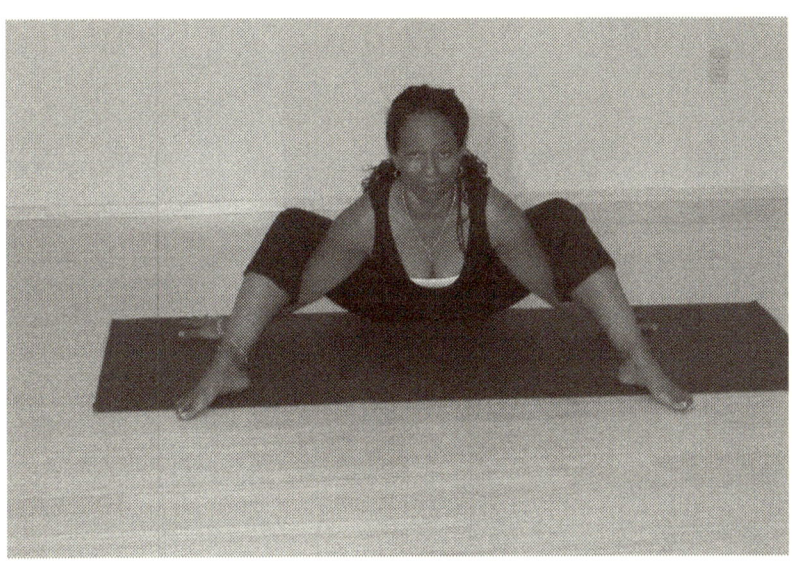

Prep for tortoise
Prep for Kurmasana

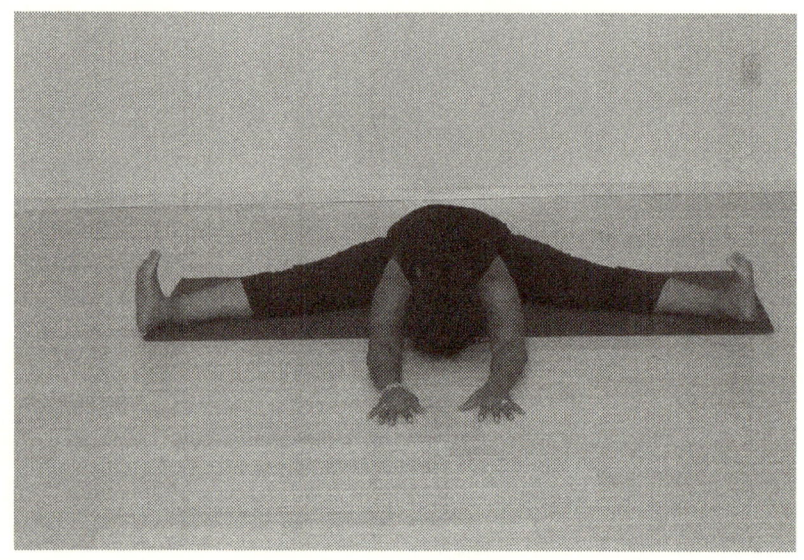

Prep for tortoise
Prep for Supta Kurmasana

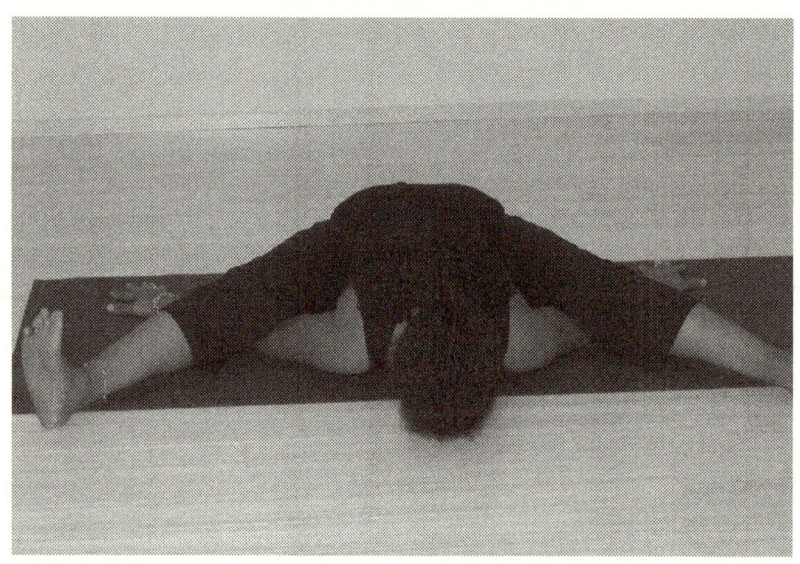

Tortoise
Supta Kurmasana

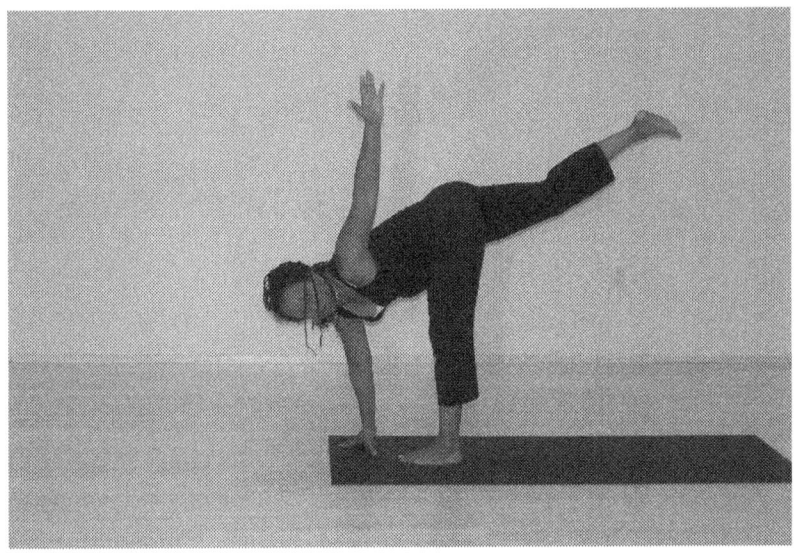

Revolved half-moon pose
Parivitta Ardha Chandrasana

Yogic Literature That Will Be Discussed

To really understand the books, I recommend Eknath Eswaran's versions (Upanishads, Gita) of the books. The commentary is easy to read. The following is just a quick overview:

- *Mahabharata*—Sanskrit epic about the dynastic struggle and civil war between the Pandavas and the Kauravas in the kingdom of Kurukshetra around the ninth century BC, and containing the text of the Bhagavad Gita, and the theology, morals, and much, much more about Hinduism and Indian history; a fascinating book for anyone interested in yoga.

- Bhagavad Gita—Sanskrit text on war on the battlefield between Krishna and Arjuna; it is a poem from the *Mahabharata* that discusses Karma, yoga, detachment, and more; I loved it, a must read.

- Vedas—Hindu scriptures (hymns); part of the Hindu Shruti; from the Vedic and Brahmanical legends; in Sanskrit *Veda* means "knowledge"; Vedas contain Surya Namascar (sun salutes) and Ayurveda.

- Upanishads—Small chapters of the Shruti with a different focus in each chapter.

A famous verse is:

Lead me from the unreal to the real
Lead me from darkness to light
Lead me from death to immortality

This verse is often chanted in Sanskrit (below) at the beginning of yoga classes.

Asatoma Sat Gamaya

Tamasoma Jyotir Gamaya

Mrityorma Amritam Gamaya

I like the Isha Upanishad, verses 15 to 18. It is recited to a dying person. It is a really good book. Read it for yourself.

Hatha Yoga Pradipika—handbook on advanced yogic practice containing several pranayama practices, mudras, kriyas, and asanas; it has more pranayama than actual asana; it only has sixteen asanas.

Yoga Sutras—*sutra* means "thread"; sutras are spoken of the most in yoga classes, in my experience; they comprise a book divided into four chapters (padas) in Sanskrit; the sutras explore yoga; the problem is that most people take them to be philosophical, and they are, but they were meant to be lived and experienced by the yogi; Patanjali organized the teaching, which prior to his organization was orally transmitted from teacher to student.

Pada one—now begins the study of yoga, what is yoga, nonattachment

Pada two—eight limbs; yama, niyamas, kleshas

Pada three—the mind fluctuations

Pada four—siddas (powers)

Patanjali's Eight Limbs of Yoga

Listed in the yoga sutras in 2:29-2:30

Yamas—moral codes, discipline, or restraints
Niyamas—cleanliness, contentment, and study; these are more personal
**Asana—the postures; detoxifies the body and prepares one to sit in meditation for long periods of time
Pranayama—breath restraint, breath control
Pratyahara—withdrawal of the senses
Dharana—concentration
Dhyana—meditation
Samadhi—bliss, enlightenment
**Asana is the third limb of yoga, but is practiced first

Yamas and Niyamas

Yamas
Ahimsa—nonviolence
Satya—truthfulness
Astyea—non-stealing
Brahmacarya—sexual abstinence, moderation
Apariygraha—greedlesness; do not take more than you need
Niyamas
Sauca—cleanliness
Santosha—contentment, happiness
Tapas—discipline
Svadhyaya—study of yourself, sacred literature
Ishvara Prandihana—surrender

Sanskrit

Sanskrit is the language yoga was originally written in. It is very tonal and resonates. It is also very easy to learn because it is so precise. It is the precursor to Latin. Should you bother to learn it?

I would learn the asana names in Sanskrit, at the very least. Most qualified teachers use the asana names in Sanskrit. So you will learn them by osmosis by just coming to class. Another reason is that, if you become a serious yogi, you will attend workshops. Most people go and see their teacher's teacher. This famous yogi will only use Sanskrit. So when the famous yogi says, "Uttakasana," you will not have to wait to see what everyone else is doing. You can move rapidly into chair pose.

I took a class through the American Sanskrit Institute by Vyass Houston. The class I took was held on the grounds of an ashram. I wanted to read the yoga sutras without the translation. I wanted to read it as it was originally written, for me. The class was excellent. They also sold tapes, books, and CDs to help with pronunciation. It is taught by chanting. You can also buy a tape of Sanskrit pronunciation from yogacenters.com.

See my new book *How to Draw Yoga Stick Figures and Learn Sanskrit Asana Names*

Mantras, Invocations, and Chants

- Mantras are phrases that are repeated in meditation, or used for a period of time to bring about a desired change.

- Traditionally, mantras are repeated 125,000 times. If you did it twice a day for thirty minutes each time it could be done in four months. Mantras can also be written or taped. Here are some of my favorites:

Om. Primordial sound with which the universe was created
Om mani padme hum. Jewel in the lotus heart
Ahum Prema. I am divine love
Tatwan Asi. You are what you seek

Gayatri Mantra
Om bhur bhuvah svaha
tat savitur varenyam
bargo devasya dhimahi
dhiyo yonah prachodayat
We honor the divine spirit
that pervades all realms of existence:
the Earth, atmosphere, and heavens.

May that most brilliant divine light
Ignorance
And illuminate our consciousness
That we might realize our goodness,
Our oneness with all.

Lokaha Samasta Sukhino Bhavantu
May all being everywhere be happy and free

Shanti, Shanti, Shanti
Peace, peace, peace

Invocations are used to create an atmosphere or set the tone for yogic practice. Anusara yoga has an invocation; Ashtanga yoga also has one. There are many others. Sometimes invocations honor the gurus (teachers, masters) that have come before us. You can purchase a CD with chants, mantras, and invocations. I find chanting CDs very nice. I listen to them in my car sometimes.

Anusara Invocation

Sanskrit

Namah Shivaya Gurave
Saccidananda Murtaye
Nisprapancaya Shantaya
Niralambaya Tejase

Translation

I offer myself to the Light, who is the True Teacher
within and without (the teacher of all teachers),
Who assumes the forms of
Reality, Consciousness and Bliss,
Who is never absent and is full of peace,
Independent in its existence,
It is the vital essence of illumination.

Chants or kirtan (chanting) can be used with any phrase or word; there are several chants.
Below is a chant to Shiva.

Shiva Bolo:

Bolo Bolo Sabmila Bolo Om Namah Shivaya. Namah Parvati Pataye Hara Hara Hara Hara Mahadev. Shiva Shiva Shankara Shiva Om Namah Shivaya. Om Namah Shivaya. Bom Bom Bolo Shiva Shiva Shankara. Shiva Shiva Shankara Shiva Shiva Shankara. Hara Hara Shambo Shiva. bolo.

What Is Ayurveda?

Ayurveda is the science of life. Imagine a book (Vedas) older than the Bible that had information like the Bible, and also had health information such as how to stay healthy (i.e., how to keep your health), and what to do for certain medical conditions (i.e., how to rejuvenate the body with Panchakarma). Ayurvedic practitioners work all over the world. Listings are available at http://www.ayurveda.com.

Treatment is based on your dosha. This is similar to your body personality type (ectomorph, mesomorph, endomorph). Treatment includes what types of food to eat, what climates are best, which seasons are best for your body type, and so forth.

Ayurveda has five elements. They are:

- Space
- Air
- Fire
- Water
- Earth

I am not an ayurvedic expert, but I do practice ayurveda, and this is just a basic overview

These elements create the body types(doshas)

- Vata—space and air
- Pitta—fire and water
- Kapha—water and earth

You can also be a combination of all three or two of them.

- Vata people—resourceful, creative, very active, even fidgety, wavy curly hair, dry skin, thin, not good with money
- Too much vata—you become spacey, irresponsible; you are not grounded
- Pitta people—fiery tempers, passionate, grounded, muscular, ambitious, and intense
- Too much pitta—frightening tempers, overly judgmental
- Kapha people—large-boned, forgiving, oily skin, funny, may have a weight problem
- Too much Kapha—greedy, selfish, controlling

These elements of ayurveda and the doshas correlate with yoga in the following ways:

- Space—Dristi (gazing)
- Air—Pranayama (breathing)
- Fire—Bhandas (locks)
- Water—Vinyasa (flow)
- Earth—Asana (yogic poses)

Is Yoga a Religion?

I am asked this question a lot. Yesterday someone said to me "I am a Christian can I do yoga?" The answer was Yes! No, yoga is not a religion, but it is a lifestyle. It does come out of the Hindu religion. Hinduism and yoga originated in India. Yoga may be far older, but is generally seen as an outgrowth of Samkhya, which is the oldest orthodox philosophical system in Hinduism. Yoga is a philosophy of thinking and mythology; it combines asana, meditation, and pranayama. Some yoga practitioners follow a strict ethical system, including such aspects as vegetarianism, celibacy, and the elements from a code known as the Yamas. Yoga may enhance religious or spiritual practices, whatever they may be. The majority of people who take classes, and the teachers who teach it in the United States are not Hindu.

After people begin taking classes on a regular basis, they generally start to have more energy, sleep better, and they discover their back is not as bad as it once was. Yoga is a philosophy that encourages positive changes. When I began taking yoga classes, I felt so good. I did not want to undo the benefits I had just received. I ate better; I no longer had my nightly glass of wine. I slept better. These changes became larger after I became a vegetarian in 1988, then a raw foodist in 1999. I changed to organic food and juice. Diet is only one small aspect of how my life has changed. These changes happened in every area of my life. It was a lifestyle change that revolved around yoga.

Personal Practice

What makes a personal practice?

Find the right time each day set aside a personal space to do your practice. I have a yoga/meditation/office. Just walking into this room is relaxing. Practice every day, whether you feel like it or not. In the morning, I hear a lot of people say they are rushed to get to work. Others feel stiff, which would make it uncomfortable. In the evening you are limited by what you can do before bedtime. Some asanas are energizing, and sleep would be difficult. Find the time that works best for you.

Buy an inexpensive kitchen timer to set to hold poses for a minute or two. (Only hold the last few poses longer after you are warmed up.) Hold longer on the tight side to increase flexibility.

Have a plan. Choose asanas that you want to go into more fully or in which you are interested.

Do about fifteen minutes a day, and gradually increase the time by five minutes each week, until you have reached thirty to forty-five minutes of asana, depending on your schedule. And do from ten to fifteen minutes of relaxation at the end. You can just lie down. Once you have established a regular practice, incorporate Pranayama and meditation in any order you prefer.

A good warm-up would be Surya Namascar (sun salutation) followed by standing asanas, balance asanas, and seated asanas. Always throw in something you love, and something you dislike. What you dislike most you probably need most. As most of us avoid the things we dislike.

Hereafter is another article I wrote for my Web site (www.lotuslore.com). This also works to begin a personal practice. Try both and decide which you prefer to begin your personal practice.

The Fast Yoga Practice

Have you ever had a morning during which you could not do your full yoga practice? This happens to me on a weekly basis almost. I have an early morning appointment that completely throws off my sadhana (spiritual practice). On days that I am not rushed, I meditate for thirty minutes, do pranayama (breathing practice) for twenty minutes, and engage in a thirty- to forty-minute yoga practice, followed by affirmations. I feel centered when I begin my day this way. Unfortunately, it is not always possible. So what do you do?

Embrace a fifteen- to twenty-minute practice. I have suggested this to my students who have told me they don't have time, don't know where to start, and so forth. This is a great way to begin your yoga practice if you do not currently have one. Just break everything up into five-minute increments:

- Five minutes of breathing

- Five minutes of yoga

- Five minutes of meditation

- Five minutes of affirmation, or reading sacred text

Change the order around to suit your needs. If you are not sure, just do two consecutive days of each, and decide which order you prefer. Sometimes it is good to mix it up. Change is good.

This will balance your day in ways you cannot imagine. The day is better for me when I do sadhana. I feel better, and I notice that I am more optimistic. I did meditate, breathe, and do yoga. Even this little bit of yoga makes a big difference in my day. Later, if you have time, you can do a little more, but it is not necessary. If you have the time, fine. If you do not have the time, fine. Yoga is all about being flexible, which applies to your schedule as well as your mind.

The fast yoga practice also works if you are sick. While recovering from a recent sinus infection, I skipped the breathing, did the rest of the practice, and my five minutes of yoga was relaxation only. I propped myself with bolsters, and

I felt renewed when I was done! It made me feel so much better. Try it; judge for yourself. Twenty minutes of practice is better than no practice at all.

Shavasana

Shavasana literally means "corpse pose."

Shavasana is the practice at the end of yoga class. It is when you do nothing and just relax. It can last anywhere from five to twenty minutes. Most new students have a difficult time relaxing. They open their eyes; some even get up and leave early, which is worse. When you leave early, the noise may disturb other students. Relaxation is very important. Very few people actually do it. Relaxation slows your nervous system down, releases stress, and slows your thought process. Shavasana is what allows your body to take in the yoga you just did. Your body did the asana, now it needs to absorb it, and rest and relaxation is how that is done.

Yoga Nidra

Yoga nidra is yogic sleep. It will normally be a class. You are not supposed to sleep during yoga nidra. Yoga nidra is yogic sleep. It is more relaxing than Shavasana. Several phrases will be repeated during yoga nidra ("I am awake; I am aware; I am practicing yoga nidra."). Directions are given to go throughout your entire body, to rest your limbs, organs, and your entire body, to rejuvenate your whole body. If you have the opportunity, attend yoga nidra. The goal is not to sleep, but you probably will; most people do in my experience.

Classes I Like

Place
Time
Day/Date
Phone number
Instructor
What I like

Place
Time
Day/Date
Phone number
Instructor
What I like

Place
Time
Day/Date
Phone number
Instructor
What I like

Place
Time
Day/Date
Phone number
Instructor
What I like

Classes I Like

Place
Time
Day/Date
Phone number
Instructor
What I like

Place
Time
Day/Date
Phone number
Instructor
What I like

Place
Time
Day/Date
Phone number
Instructor
What I like

Place
Time
Day/Date
Phone number
Instructor
What I like

Classes/Workshop Notes
Information on workshops or
classes attended recently

Classes/Workshop Notes
Information on workshops or classes attended recently

Classes/Workshop Notes
Information on workshops or
classes attended recently

Classes/Workshop Notes
Information on workshops or
classes attended recently

Telephone Book

Name
Home phone
Cell phone
Work phone
Address
E-mail

Name
Home phone
Cell phone
Work phone
Address
E-mail

Name
Home phone
Cell phone
Work phone
Address
E-mail

Name
Home phone
Cell phone
Work phone
Address
E-mail

Name
Home phone
Cell phone
Work phone
Address
E-mail

Name
Home phone
Cell phone
Work phone
Address
E-mail

Name
Home phone
Cell phone
Work phone
Address
E-mail

Name
Home phone
Cell phone
Work phone
Address
E-mail
Phone Book
Name
Home phone
Cell phone
Work phone
Address
E-mail

Name
Home phone
Cell phone
Work phone
Address
E-mail

Name
Home phone
Cell phone
Work phone
Address
E-mail

Name
Home phone
Cell phone
Work phone
Address
E-mail

Recommended reading list I created as librarian for the Suncoast Yoga Teachers Association

For a well-rounded yoga education

Yoga for Body, Breath, and Mind, Mohan
Heart of Yoga, Deskkchar
Happy Yoga, Steve Ross
Yoga for Common Ailments, Dr. Monro, Dr. Nagarathna, Dr. Nagendra
Yoga Mala, Sri K. Jois, Sri K. Pattabhi Jois
Ashtanga Yoga, John Scott
Yoga Practice Manual, David Swenson
Light on Yoga, B. K. S. Iyengar
Light on Pranayama, B. K. S. Iyengar
Autobiography of a Yogi, Paramahansa Yogananda
Teach Yourself Sanskrit, complete course for beginners
Yoga Sutras, any version, although I recommend *Yoga Sutra Workbook*, American Sanskrit Institute
Dictionary of Sanskrit Yoga Asana Names, Integral Yoga Institute
Shivananda Companion to Yoga
Healing Path of Yoga, Nischala Joy Devi
Yoga the Iyengar Way, Silva, Mira & Shyam Mehta
Living Yoga, Christy Turlington
Upanishads, Bhagvdad Gita, Dhamapada, all Eknath Easwaran versions
Hatha Yoga Pradipika, Shivananda version
Meditation, Eknath Easwaran
Full Catastrophe Living, Jon Kabat Zinn
Moving into Stillness, Eric Shiffman
Yoga Poetry of the Body, Rodney Yee
Kundalini Yoga Shakti Parwha Kaur Khasla
Eight Human Talents, Gurmukh
Jivamukti Yoga, Sharon Gannon, David Life

Power Yoga, Beyond Power Yoga, Berryl Bender Birch
Yoga for the Three Stages of Life, Srivatsa Ramaswami
Bikrams Beginning Yoga Class
Ayurveda, Dr. Viriod Verma
Ayurveda & Panchakarma, Saril Vijoshi, MD
Om Yoga, Cindi Lee
Asana Pranayama and Mudra Banda & Yoga Nidra, Swami Satananda Saraswati
Partner Yoga, Carroll and Kimata
Yoga for Wellness, Gary Kraftsow
Trail Guide to the Body
Anatonomy of Movement, Cladis Germaine
Play of Consciousness, Swami Muktananda
Rest, Relax, and Renew, Judith Lassiter

Notes

Notes

Visit my Web sites
www.lotuslore.com and www.innerpeaceyoga.org

978-0-595-35924-0
0-595-35924-8

www.ingramcontent.com/pod-product-compliance
Lightning Source LLC
Chambersburg PA
CBHW020341290526
45785CB00005B/2128